Introd...
the Carni...

A Beginner's Guide to Understanding the Health Benefits of a Meat-Only Diet

W.M. O'Brien

Disclaimer Notice:

Please note the information contained within this document is for educational and entertainment purposes only. All effort has been executed to present accurate, up to date, reliable, complete information. No warranties of any kind are declared or implied. Readers acknowledge that the author is not engaged in the rendering of legal, financial, medical or professional advice. The content within this book has been derived from various sources. Please consult a licensed professional before attempting any techniques outlined in this book.

By reading this document, the reader agrees that under no circumstances is the author responsible for any losses, direct or indirect, that are incurred as a result of the use of the information contained within this document, including, but not limited to, errors, omissions, or inaccuracies.

Table of Contents

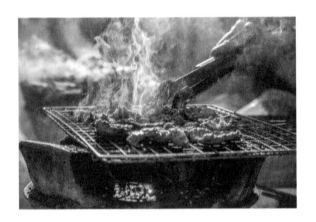

Introduction

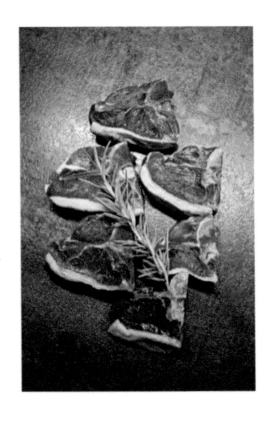

Tens of thousands or even millions of years ago, humankind were carnivores. Arguably, some—Canada's and Greenland's Inuit—still are (Saladino, 2022).

While this traditional perception of the "caveman" and their diets has met challenges, the prevailing discussion on the topic seems to leave room on the omnivore scale for degrees, from the so-called "hypercarnivore" to something closer to the condition of most of the modern world's population (Parsons, 2019; Roxby, 2010; McAuliffe, 2021b).

Why is this important? It isn't, unless you're an anthropologist or—far more likely—you picked up this book to learn about the potential benefits of a carnivorous diet and how it could help you.

First, however, you should know what this book is not: It isn't a cookbook— there are lots of those—nor will it hype these benefits to the exclusion of every other supposed "fad" diet. Like others, the carnivore diet has a purpose—which is primarily to support weight loss and probably how you've heard of it, and so it's up to you, the reader, to determine if this diet is right for you.

To assist you in this decision, I will explain what the carnivore diet is—specifically, what foods are and aren't permitted; its benefits; and how it differs from diets such as the ketogenic (keto) diet and others. Without getting too clinical, I'll also offer some primary nutritional information, a few typical daily meal plans, and an overview of its potential risks, in addition to the latest science-based data.

Note: To assist the reader with perhaps unfamiliar terms, certain words will be *italicized* upon first use in this book; these, and others that you may have come across elsewhere in your research or daily life, are included in the "Glossary" with a brief definition for clarity in context.

The Carnivore Diet

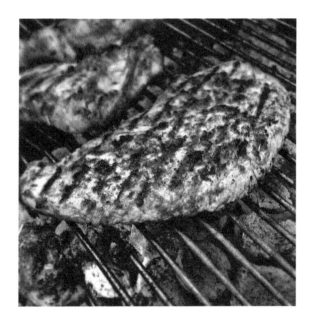

As you might imagine, the *carnivore diet* is made up almost exclusively of meat and animal products—for example fish and shellfish; beef; pork; poultry; organ meats (kidney and liver); plus fats such as butter and lard. Some may include certain dairy products—for example, eggs, milk, and cheese—but all exclude anything plant-based—that is, cereals and grains and their derivatives, including flour and cornmeal; nuts and seeds; legumes (peas, lentils, and so on); soy; plus all vegetables and fruits. In other words, nothing that doesn't come from an animal—making it the opposite of a *vegan* diet (check the "Differences" section for more).

While the inclusion of "healthier" choices of fish and leaner white meats (skinless chicken) is generally okay for variety, the point of the carnivore diet is to get a higher fat intake along with protein, so frequent consumption of these is counterproductive—more details to follow.

Importantly, almost all beverages are excluded from the carnivore diet. These obviously include fruit or veggie juices, but also [*gasp!*] coffee and tea, as well as alcoholic ones, since virtually all beer, wine, and spirits are made from grains or other plants such as fruit, or honey. Speaking of honey, sweeteners are a no-no as well, including: honey; sugar; corn or maple syrup; and the like.

Thus, plain water appears to be your only choice here—but note that, unless you're perhaps an elite athlete (Henry Ford Health, 2017), virtually all health professionals promote plain, unflavored, and noncarbonated water over any other drink; it's unmatched in providing hydration and contains no calories (UC Davis, 2022; Government of Canada, 2021; Centers for Disease Control and Prevention [CDC], n.d.-b). Even so, while scientific data appear scanty, many proponents tout the increased sense of hydration felt by adding Himalayan pink salt to make sole water (Leonard, 2018; Streit, 2019; WebMD Editorial Contributors, 2022; Millard, 2022).

So, no loss, right? Then again, an older study may say otherwise (Maughan et al., 2015). Oh dear. I'll have more to say on these conflicting opinions later.

While proteins (see "Dietary Basics" section) include legumes, nuts, and seeds, as a strict carnivore these are not permitted. However, certain dairy proteins such as kefir (thick yogurt) and cheese may be allowed on your carnivore diet plan or per your preference (see also "My Two Cents" and "Conclusion"). There are choices here too: For one, it promotes hard cheeses like parmesan or cheddar as having higher protein—and *sodium*—while being lower in *lactose* when compared to soft cheeses like brie (McAuliffe, 2022b).

Another caveat regarding dairy before we move on: There is apparently a difference between what are referred to as *A1* and *A2* dairy proteins (Kruszelnicki, 2018), collectively called *casein*, although no conclusive proof exists regarding which might cause problems (Pal et al., 2015). Despite some anecdotal reports of sensitivity to one or the other (Saladino, 2021), the reader may again wish to experiment with this choice. However, be advised that problems with dairy products can be caused by lactose, not necessarily casein (Pal et al., 2015).

While considering meat, keep in mind that many—especially *processed* such as wieners, sausages, and premade hamburger patties, plus so-called "delicatessen meats"—may contain *binders* or *fillers* that are plant-based, such as breadcrumbs, flour, maltodextrin (a starch-based food *additive*), soy, or oatmeal. If your goal is to eliminate these food groups, be aware that some proponents of the carnivore diet recommend against processed meats anyway (Sanchez, 2020).

There is also the consideration of "how much," as in, to eat. This depends in part on your goal, and recommended serving sizes vary, but for weight loss at least one website recommends a ratio of 1 g (.035 oz) of protein per pound (2.2 kilograms) of your body-weight goal, to which you "add high quality animal fat... until satiety. This will usually end up being about a 1:1 protein to fat ratio in terms of grams. Remember that 1 pound of meat has about 100g [3.527 oz] of protein" (Saladino, 2022, para. 12).

This "until satiety" seems a reasonable statement, to which I'll return later.

Differences

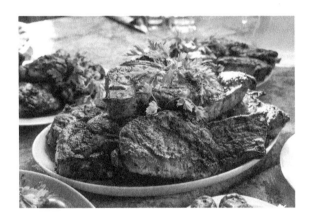

While the purpose of this book isn't to cover other diets, I will provide a few very brief distinctions from other popular diets to differentiate with the intent of helping to clarify your choices.

The carnivore diet differs from a ketogenic or the Atkins diet in that the latter restrict carbohydrates in varying degrees, while carnivores attempt to eliminate them completely.

The carnivore diet is also not like Jenny Craig or WeightWatchers, in that the former is self-managed and -directed, while the latter groups provide outside coaching and support, along with meal plans, recipes, and so forth.

To conclude this section, I'll give the reader an abbreviated overview of the dozens and dozens of others, starting with the California, Sonoma, and Mediterranean diets; these are apparently just variants on one another, based on locally available foods and cultural preferences. The dietary approaches to stop hypertension (DASH) and Flexitarian diet are primarily for diabetics; Mediterranean-DASH intervention for neurodegenerative delay (MIND) and Dr. Weil's anti-inflammatory diets are plant-based; paleo, Keyto—different from but similar to keto—and Optavia are high in protein.

Even so, there appears to be lots of crossover between most of these. Moreover, some, like the Mayo Clinic diet, are accompanied by complex plans and restrictions, so we won't go any further. But I'm sure you'll find a book or two on any of them if you're interested!

Dietary Basics

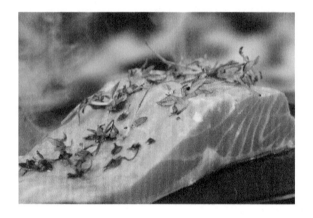

To understand the potential benefits of the carnivore diet, a very basic comprehension of *dietetics* and nutrition seems necessary.

First, you've likely heard that food comes in *groups*: grains, aka starches; proteins; fruits and vegetables; fats and oils; and perhaps "other." The latter group may include certain items that are considered additives or flavorings—for example, salt, or else those that are *empty* of *calories* such as candy and soda, perhaps even extending to all sweets: cake, pie, cookies, and so on. However, for our purposes, these aren't animal-based anyway, and therefore excluded in a strict carnivore diet. Yes, you heard right: *No dessert for you*, unless you make it out of an animal product like ice cream, skipping ingredients such as vanilla and sugar. Also, although it restricts herbs and spices, see my thoughts on these and other restrictions later on in the book.

Proteins, Carbs, and the Rest... Oh My!

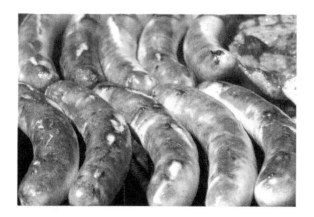

Meat, as you probably already know, is primarily a protein. Grains are key sources of carbohydrates (carbs), and vegetables and fruits provide various *nutrients*, as well as, to a lesser extent, carbs.

Foods other than meat and fish contain varying amounts of carbohydrates, the primary source of the body's "fuel" (covered later). They also provide variable amounts of *minerals* and *vitamins*, essential nutrients for human health. Since many of these might be found in but a single group—or only in trace amounts in some groups— restricting one or more food groups necessarily limits the intake of some nutrients. For example, Vitamin C, which is primarily found in fruits and vegetables, is critical to avoid symptoms of *scurvy* and will need to be acquired through dietary supplements like over-the-counter multivitamins and similar means. So, if you're opposed to putting "synthetic" substances in your body—

albeit there are many so-called "organic alternatives"—then be advised.

To conclude this section, even though various jurisdictions' labels and classifications of the described food groups differ and often change, the basics remain the same, namely that carbs are what is metabolized or "burned" as fuel by the body first, followed by fat, and then protein.

This fact forms the basic premise of the carnivore diet, specifically, that it burns fat. I hear you: "Yes, but will it burn *mine*?" Read on to learn about some more potential benefits as well.

The Benefits

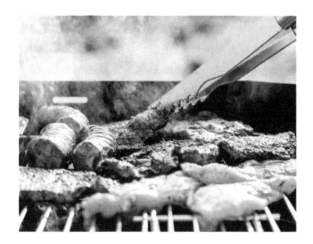

Since burning fat is the given primary goal of weight-loss diets, including the carnivore diet, if that's your intended purpose (see later for other possible reasons), getting to this state instead of burning carbohydrates, called *ketosis*, is easier when your only intake is protein and fat.

As an all-protein eater, being a carnivore offers the side benefit of high *satiety*; that is, the feeling of fullness from protein—and fat—is experienced much sooner and for longer than that which would be provided by a similar caloric intake of carbs. And this sensation, in turn, naturally inhibits snacking, which as we know is a key factor that hinders weight loss. Note that some carnivore diet meal plans incorporate snacks while others do not (more later regarding this discrepancy too).

While testimonials exist that advocate relief of myriad symptoms caused by depression and anxiety; arthritis; and many others (Hamblin, 2018; McAuliffe,

2021a), scientific evidence for these claims is still lacking (Bianchetti, 2021), albeit the early hue and cry against the practice appears to be decelerating (see "The Science").

Still, it probably goes without saying that the carnivore diet, by excluding *fiber* (see "The Risks") and *gluten*, may benefit people with such *sensitivities* or even diseases such as *celiac disease*. Similarly, those with a lactose *intolerance* or sensitivity can avoid symptoms by excluding dairy products, while keeping eggs on their menu if they so choose.

The Science

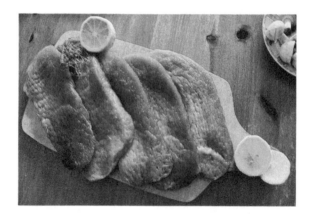

I've mentioned that the hard science is still lacking for almost all purported benefits of the carnivore diet. What's out there is largely anecdotal, but this doesn't mean you shouldn't try it if you have conditions such as those mentioned previously; just be aware of the risks (see "The Risks"), while considering the following.

First, however, at least some websites recommend getting your blood tested before starting this diet, and continuing to do so regularly during use, to screen for potential higher-than-normal risks (again, "The Risks") for conditions such as high cholesterol and diabetes.

The most recent hard science data as of this writing is from the same study published on both the ScienceDirect and the National Library of Medicine websites (Lennerz et al., 2021). Although this report seems trustworthy, there are a lot of qualifiers, including how some subjects reported that they consumed other than meat, and more than one-third denied the use of supplements. According to other data, this last appears risky (see "The Risks").

But before I get to the risks of the carnivore diet, I want to briefly return to the opening statement of this book regarding ancient humanity, specifically regarding *Neanderthals* and the Inuit culture. It needs to be stated that *metabolic*—perhaps including cultural—differences are likely factors in being able to consume a nearly all-meat diet safely or comfortably. According to several studies I found—even one from going on 90 years ago, but in my opinion still relevant, by Rabinowitch et al. (1936)—a metabolic predisposition toward consumption of a given food type is almost assuredly a factor in one's ability to do so (Munch-Andersen et al., 2012; Naqitarvik et al., 2022).

Thus, if you suspect you might have Inuit—and most of us have Neanderthal *DNA* (Teague & McRae, n.d.)—genes in your makeup, you may already have an advantage toward adopting this diet!

The Risks

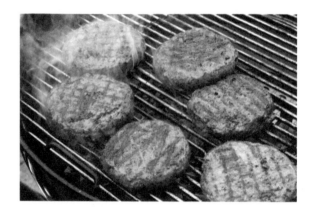

Alas, the problems.

Aside from potential vitamin and mineral deficiencies, boredom appears to perhaps be the primary "risk" of a meat-only diet; there are only so many varieties and cuts that are done so many ways, and if you can't use seasonings... However, that's where a dedicated cookbook may come in handy—a quick online search produced hundreds of thousands of hits.

When it comes to using seasonings, salt is usually okayed and pepper is often allowed, but herbs and spices appear to be largely excluded along with sauces and other condiments. So, the blandness and monotony of different types and cuts of meat even prepared in a variety of ways—sautéing, boiling, roasting, grilling, and so on—may be an issue for you, unless you're a creative cook!

Nonetheless, the more serious risk, aside from the aforementioned, is the diet's lack of fiber; a diet lacking in fiber, as you likely know, can lead to constipation and more serious problems. Conversely, meat and fat are identified with a higher likelihood of experiencing symptoms of constipation (National Institute on Aging, n.d.; Slattery, n.d.). Still, people differ; many —even not considering those with an *inflammatory bowel disease* (IBS)—will profess more difficulties ingesting fiber or gluten than red meat, so the absence of the former will obviously aid such persons. Again, choice and your personal circumstances become relative and vital.

Before moving on—sorry, that wasn't a pun, honest!—it's further important to note that other factors play a role, sometimes significant, in contributing to constipation: a lack of regular exercise, pregnancy, plus many over-the-counter and prescription medications which can cause such symptoms. So, again, "Your results may vary."

Also worthy to heed is a potential loss of "good bacteria." As we know, many diverse bacteria are required in the gut and intestines to digest food, and so the loss of some can be problematic (Rinninella et al., 2019; Harvard University, n.d.-b).

Additionally, if you use salt to enhance flavors—perhaps overdoing it in lieu of other condiments, as one might imagine —you risk elevating your sodium levels, which can have myriad consequences, from headaches to heart and kidney disease (CDC, n.d.-a).

Plus, we all know about heart disease and *saturated fats* (American Heart Association, n.d.), which will almost certainly be increased on this diet; thus, the caveat earlier about getting frequent blood tests.

Finally, if you choose to make processed meats part of your carnivore diet, keep in mind that these carry risks aside from those mentioned, such as high *nitrates*, a suspected *carcinogen* and contributor to heart disease and diabetes (Gallagher, 2015; National Cancer Institute, 2022). Then again, certain plants have naturally occurring nitrates and, consequently, *nitrites* (Chazelas, 2022; Newman, 2022); so, once more, be informed.

Typical Meal Plans

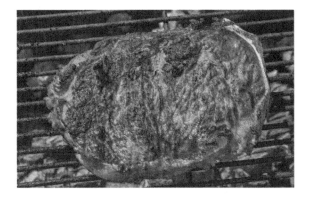

A typical carnivore-diet meal plan might include the following:

Meal	Day 1	Day 2	Day 3	Day 4
Breakfast	Eggs, fried in butter or bacon fat; bacon	Gruyére cheese omelet; pork sausage	Eggs, scrambled in butter or bacon fat; fried ham	N.Y. strip steak and fried eggs
Lunch	Baked chicken breasts; cottage cheese	Assorted cold cuts; kefir	Sauteed chicken strips (NO breading or coating); hard-boiled eggs	Grilled salmon filet; side of sauteed chicken livers
Dinner	Porterhouse beef steak; side of sardines	Braised pork chops; cheddar cheese	Roast beef (opt.: gravy thickened with ghee*); side of sautéed shrimp	Broiled pork steak under melted brie cheese

*Clarified butter; see "Glossary." Note that substitute thickeners such as xanthan gum, tapioca, arrowroot, and so forth are not allowed on the carnivore diet, as they are all made from plants.

As indicated, meals don't have to always be hot; cold cuts, such as pastrami, bologna, and more are for some people ideal luncheon meats (but see elsewhere re: caveats against inclusion, such as health risks and potential fillers). You can alternatively precook beef or chicken strips, as only two examples, and have them cold for lunch the next day.

Moreover, as you can probably extrapolate from the table, you can substitute various cuts of meat; the given examples don't have to repeat endlessly! Try incorporating chicken, turkey, or beef sausage; a wide variety of other fish and seafood, if you're not allergic; a filet mignon steak wrapped in LOTS of bacon; liver or kidneys—from chicken, lamb, or beef—for your breakfast meat or for a supper meal; ground or shredded textures; and so on. There are options, so get creative—or get hold of some cookbooks!

My Two Cents

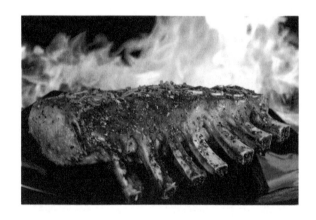

I would now like to offer a few opinions and recommendations, based on my background and further research.

First, to me, excluding tea and coffee seems redundant; you get no actual calories from either—unless, obviously, you add cream or sugar. Moreover, while they do contain some toxins, they overwhelmingly contain beneficial *polyphenols*. Perhaps most importantly, for many humans, a nice hot cup of coffee or tea at the right time is simply relaxing if not downright necessary! Finally, some websites cited herein promote hot beverages, albeit the only one typically recommended appears to be bone broth—or presumably warm milk. Yech, how dull!

Another observation is that there seem to be a lot of self-serving websites out there, some with downright dangerous if not simply spurious claims. At least one states that coffee contains carcinogens and "pesticides and herbicides that can be extremely toxic and cause serious long-term health problems" (Le, 2022, "2. Coffee," point 4). Excuse me? Ever heard of organic coffee, or doing research to back up such suspect claims (Sakamoto et al., 2012; Government of Canada, 2018; Harvard University, n.d.-a)? But when a website can't spell or use correct grammar, I dismiss it immediately, despite any claims of having a PhD: "Phytate. Why some animals can handly phytate, humans can't" (Le, 2022, "3. Tea," point 4).

That's just one example, and so I strongly caution the reader to take with a grain of salt, if not prohibited on your diet, any assertions made by websites other than governmental or institutional sites—that is, universities or other bona fides, even those cited here.

Thus, like coffee and tea, why exclude alcohol? I'm not considering the negative health benefits of overconsumption here; that's not the scope of this book. Precious few "nutrients," especially carbs, are extruded from grains or grapes during processing and fermentation, with fewer still left to pass along to you upon ingestion. Furthermore, wine—at least red—for one, though not conclusively proven, appears even beneficial (Mayo Clinic Staff, 2022a).

Even so, besides drunkenness and alcoholism, some authors allude to other downsides to alcohol, namely, that it's a psychoactive drug and that "your body processes alcohol differently. Alcohol interferes with fat metabolism, increases weight gain, and can get you drunk faster, more intensely, and leave you with worse hangovers" (Le, 2022; McAuliffe, 2022a, "Dr. Kiltz's Bottom Line: Carnivore Diet and Alcohol," para. 3). But I see little hard evidence for these specific assertions (Rehm, 2011; CDC, n.d.-a). Instead, in a bit, see what Oscar Wilde has to say.

Without turning this book into a rant against the carnivore diet—far from it! Personally, I'm left with other questions.

For example, I wonder about vinegars—and there are *many* varieties, all of which I won't list here. For our purposes, take plain white vinegar: It's made up of acetic acid (chemical formula CH_3COOH) and water, so presumably it's acceptable on the carnivore diet as a rather basic "condiment." But almost all other vinegars are made with barley, fruit, or rice, so they're presumably forbidden. Still, my point remains in regards to the amount of nutrients, especially injurious ones, absorbable through, say, a few sprinkles of balsamic vinegar on your sautéed shrimp.

As Oscar Wilde (n.d.) says, "Everything in moderation." So, once you've chosen to adopt a carnivore diet, I hereby offer my suggestion to gradually introduce yourself to it. Many of the sources I've already referenced, as well as others (Woods, 2022), recommend such a progressed approach—for example, not completely cutting out greens, dairy, or anything else all at once—for your body may experience withdrawal-like symptoms, if not go into shock when Friday Pizza Night comes around!

But seriously, starting something new can be scary enough without trying to overdo it, so go slowly. And, incidentally, the same sources caution you not to expect results for several weeks, so don't fret and burn this book—although I don't know if ereaders are flammable, I wouldn't experiment anyway—when you're not losing a pound, or whatever, per week.

Also keep in mind that the main point of eating—other than fueling the body, naturally, and for social reasons—is, after all, to feel full and satisfied, so when considering all of the foregoing along with portion sizes and how often and when to eat, go with whatever suits your lifestyle and goals.

Finally, as with starting any diet or exercise program, do consult with a doctor or registered dietitian beforehand.

Conclusion

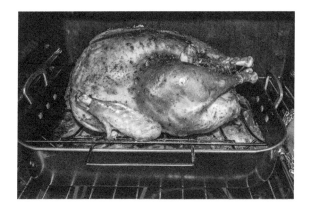

Despite the contradictory claims and evidence, I hope you have been able to glean a little clarity from this book. As I've tried to emphasize, your choices are what make a "diet." Whether you're looking for weight loss, relief of unfriendly gastrointestinal symptoms, or want to try out some of the claims of respite from other reported adverse conditions, then go for it! As with any diet, your personal modifications and preferences, as well as your metabolism, play a role; you can choose to be very restrictive in eliminating everything not rigorously "carnivore," or not so much.

You are an adult, after all.

Glossary

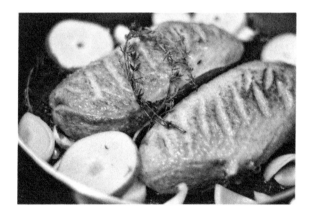

A1/A2: Types of dairy protein; mostly anecdotal evidence suggests some people may find A2 dairy products easier to absorb, although they're generally more expensive—where they can be found.

Additive: Used in food, a substance intended to boost flavor or act as a preservative; most often chemical and not organic.

Binder/Filler: A substance that adds bulk to a food and/or binds ingredients together, commonly used in sausages, delicatessen meats, and so forth.

Calorie (Cal): Unit of measure for the body's consumption of food; also, kilocalorie (kCal). Some countries use kilojoules (kJ).

Carcinogen: Something that can cause or contribute to causing cancer.

Casein: A dairy protein.

Celiac disease: An autoimmune condition where the small intestines cannot process gluten.

Dietetics: The study or science of diet and nutrition.

Deoxyribonucleic acid (DNA): The double helix making up the genome of every creature, discovered by Watson and Crick.

Empty calories: Foodstuffs providing little nutritional or caloric value that still provide satiety.

Fiber (soluble, insoluble): Soluble fiber absorbs water and slows digestion; insoluble fiber adds bulk to the stool and assists food in passing more quickly through the digestive system.

Filler/Binder: See *binder/filler*.

Food group: Categorizations of food types, generally: grains; meats and alternates; vegetables and fruits; dairy and alternates; fats and oils; perhaps including other. It can vary in title and designation between jurisdictions, as well as change over time.

Fructose: A natural sugar found in fruit.

Genome: Connected "strings" of DNA making up the structure of a given creature: e.g., the human genome.

Ghee: Clarified butter used in East Indian cooking.

Glucose: The sugar into which the body metabolizes food to be absorbed as "fuel." It can be artificial, as used in diabetics' injections.

Gluten: A substance found in wheat, barley, rye, et al., that many people find dietarily difficult to absorb; see *celiac* and *inflammatory bowel disease* and *inflammatory bowel syndrome* definitions.

Ketosis: The state in which the body is burning fat and/or protein rather than carbohydrates; can be entered into safely or unsafely.

Inflammatory bowel disease (IBD): Various diseases of the bowels (intestinal tract) such as Crohn's or colitis.

Intolerance: An important distinction should be made between a sensitivity (q.v.) and an intolerance or disease. Some people have minor symptoms (sensitivity) when consuming, say, gluten, while for others, these can be severe (intolerance). Only a health professional can distinguish the difference and prescribe treatment.

Irritable bowel syndrome (IBS): Distinguished from IBD, IBS can have an array of causes; see also sensitivity and intolerance.

Lactose: A natural sugar found in dairy products; many people can be sensitive or intolerant.

Legume: A member of a plant family high in protein, including peas, lentils, and beans (e.g., pinto, kidney, chickpeas or garbanzos); it is often dried, and sometimes called "pulse."

Metabolism: The intrinsic process within an individual human by which they process food or benefit—or not—from exercise (e.g., a "high-metabolism" person burns energy quickly).

Mineral: An inorganic element found in food; some are essential to human health, with iron being most commonly known.

Monounsaturated (fat or oil): Refers to natural fats found in certain plant oils, e.g. peanut, olive, safflower, sesame, and canola. See also *saturated*, *unsaturated*, *monounsaturated*, *trans*.

Neanderthal: A protohuman species; works cited herein indicate that most of us retain traces of Neanderthal DNA, which may or may not help us metabolize high-fat, high-protein diets.

Nitrate: Sodium nitrate is a chemical additive used to enhance the flavor of meat; generally harmful to human health.

Nitrite: When sodium nitrate (see *nitrate*) is consumed it's turned into a nitrite; both are almost equally harmful.

Nutrient (macro- or micro-): A substance found in food, such as minerals or vitamins, essential for human health.

Phytonutrients: Nutrients found in plants.

Polyunsaturated (fat or oil): Refers to natural fats found in certain plant oils (e.g. sunflower, corn, and soybean). See also *saturated*, *unsaturated*, *monounsaturated*, *trans*.

Processed meat: Meat that has gone through a commercial process of deboning, grinding, etc., often including the addition of spices and herbs, plus binders/fillers and other additives to make, for example, sausage or bologna.

Pulse: See *legume*.

Satiety: The feeling of fullness when eating.

Saturated (fat): Solid at room temperature; associated with LDL cholesterol, or "bad fat." See also *monounsaturated, polyunsaturated, unsaturated, trans.*

Scurvy: A disease caused primarily by a vitamin-C deficiency.

Sensitivity: See *intolerance.*

Sodium: Sodium chloride is plain table salt, but there are others—sodium nitrate, for example. While sodium is an essential nutrient, in excess—the norm for most of us—it is very harmful.

Sucrose: A natural sugar found in sugar beets or sugarcane.

Toxin: A poison.

Trans (fat): A liquid fat chemically changed into a solid, such as vegetable oil for deep frying. Trans fat is much worse for health than even saturated.

See also *monounsaturated, polyunsaturated, unsaturated.*

Unsaturated (fat): Stays liquid at room temperature; associated with HDL cholesterol, or "good fat." See also *monounsaturated, polyunsaturated, saturated, trans.*

Vitamin: A nutrient found in food; most are essential to human health.

Vegan (diet): A diet that eschews all animal products. Sometimes, it refers to a person who subscribes to this diet.

Vegetarian (diet): A diet consisting of only vegetables, fruits, and grains, albeit a "lacto-ovo vegetarian" will consume certain dairy products and eggs. Sometimes, it refers to a person who subscribes to this diet.

References

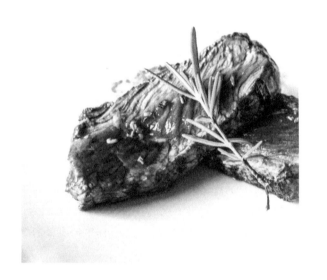

American Heart Association. (n.d.). *Saturated fat.* https://www.heart.org/en/healthy-living/healthy-eating/eat-smart/fats/saturated-fats

Bianchetti, B. (2021, September 29). *7 reported carnivore diet benefits.* People's Choice Beef Jerky. https://peopleschoicebeefjerky.com/blogs/news/carnivore-diet-benefits

Centers for Disease Control and Prevention. (n.d.-b). *Get the facts: Data and research on water consumption.* U.S. Department of Health and Human Services, National Institutes of Health. https://www.cdc.gov/nutrition/data-statistics/plain-water-the-healthier-choice.html

Centers for Disease Control and Prevention. (n.d.-c). *Sodium.* U.S. Department of Health and

Human Services, National Institutes of Health. https://www.cdc.gov/heartdisease/sodium.htm

Centers for Disease Control and Prevention. (n.d.-a). *Alcohol use and your health*. https://www.cdc.gov/alcohol/fact-sheets/alcohol-use.htm

Chazelas, E., Pierre, F., Druesne-Pecollo, N., Esseddik, Y., Szabo de Edelenyi, F., Agaesse, C., De Sa, A., Lutchia, R., Gigandet, S., Srour, B., Debras, C., Huybrechts, I., Julia, C., Kesse-Guyot, E., Allès, B., Galan, P., Hercberg, S., Deschasaux-Tanguy, M., & Touvier, M. (2022). Nitrites and nitrates from food additives and natural sources and cancer risk: Results from the NutriNet-Santé cohort. *International Journal of Epidemiology, 51*(4), 1106–1119. https://doi.org/10.1093/ije/dyac046

National Institute on Aging (n.d.). *Concerned about constipation?* U.S. Department of Health and Human Services, National Institutes of Health. https://www.nia.nih.gov/health/concerned-about-constipation

Gallagher, J. (2015, October 26). *Processed meats do cause cancer —WHO.* BBC News. https://www.bbc.com/news/health-34615621

Government of Canada. (2018, September 4). *2010–2011 pesticides in coffee, fruit juice and tea.* https://inspection.canada.ca/food-safety-for-industry/food-chemistry-and-microbiology/food-safety-testing-bulletin-and-reports/pesticides/eng/1351913846907/1351913943956

Hamblin, J. (2018, August 28). *The Jordan Peterson all-meat diet.* The Atlantic. https://

www.theatlantic.com/health/
archive/2018/08/the-peterson-
family-meat-cleanse/567613/

Harvard University. (n.d.-a). *Coffee.*
https://www.hsph.harvard.edu/
nutritionsource/food-features/
coffee/

Harvard University. (n.d.-b). *The
microbiome.* https://
www.hsph.harvard.edu/
nutritionsource/microbiome/

Government of Canada. (2021, January
26). *Make water your drink of
choice.* https://food-
guide.canada.ca/en/healthy-
eating-recommendations/make-
water-your-drink-of-choice/

Henry Ford Health Staff. (2017, October
12). *Sports drinks vs. Water:
What's the best way to hydrate?*
Henry Ford Health. https://
www.henryford.com/blog/
2017/10/sports-drinks-vs-water-
b e s t - w a y -

hydrate#:~:text=When%20it%20
comes%20to%20athletic

Hinzey, E., & Schueller, G. (2023, January 3). *U.S. news best diets: How we rated eating plans and diets.* U.S. News & World Report. https://health.usnews.com/ wellness/food/articles/how-us-news-ranks-best-diets

IARC Working Group on the Evaluation of Carcinogenic Risks to Humans. (1991). Coffee, tea, mate, methylxanthines and methylglyoxal. *International Agency for Research on Cancer, 51.* https:// www.ncbi.nlm.nih.gov/books/ NBK507034/

Kruszelnicki, K. (2018, June 18). *Dr Karl explains the difference between A1 and A2 milk.* ABC News. https://www.abc.net.au/ news/science/2018-06-19/dr-karl-a1-vs-a2-milk/

9879800#:~:text=The%20only%20difference%20between%20A1

Le, S. (2022, February 17). *Drinks on the carnivore diet: The great, the okay, and the stay-away.* All Things Carnivore. https://www.allthingscarnivore.com/drinks-on-the-carnivore-diet-the-good-the-okay-and-the-stay-away/

Lennerz, B. S., Mey, J. T., Henn, O. H., & Ludwig, D. S. (2021). Behavioral characteristics and self-reported health status among 2029 adults consuming a "carnivore diet." *Current Developments in Nutrition*, 5(12). https://doi.org/10.1093/cdn/nzab133

Leonard, J. (2018, July 30). *Does pink himalayan salt have any health benefits?* Medical News Today. https://www.medicalnewstoday.com/articles/315081

Llczbiński, P., & Bukowska, B. (2022). Tea and coffee polyphenols and their biological properties based on the latest in vitro investigations. *Industrial Crops and Products*, *175*, 114265. https://doi.org/10.1016/j.indcrop.2021.114265

Maughan, R. J., Watson, P., Cordery, P. A. A., Walsh, N. P., Oliver, S. J., Dolci, A., Rodriguez-Sanchez, N., & Galloway, S. D. R. (2015). A randomized trial to assess the potential of different beverages to affect hydration status: Development of a beverage hydration index. *The American Journal of Clinical Nutrition*, *103*(3), 717–723. https://doi.org/10.3945/ajcn.115.114769

Mayo Clinic Staff. (2022b, February 23). *Trans fat: Double trouble for your heart*. Mayo Clinic. https://www.mayoclinic.org/diseases-conditions/high-blood-

cholesterol/in-depth/trans-fat/
art-20046114

Mayo Clinic Staff. (2022a, January 14).
*Red wine and resveratrol: Good
for your heart?* Mayo Clinic.
https://www.mayoclinic.org/
diseases-conditions/heart-
disease/in-depth/red-wine/
art-20048281#:~:text=Red%20w
ine%2C%20in%20moderation%2
C%20has

McAuliffe, L. (2021a, May 27). *9
carnivore diet benefits and how
to get them.* Doctor Kiltz. https://
www.doctorkiltz.com/carnivore-
diet-benefits/

McAuliffe, L. (2021b, December 31).
*What did cavemen eat? Lots of
meat, new study reveals.* Doctor
Kiltz. https://
www.doctorkiltz.com/what-
cavemen-eat/

McAuliffe, L. (2022a, August 11).
Carnivore diet and alcohol:

What you need to know. Doctor Kiltz. https://www.doctorkiltz.com/carnivore-diet-and-alcohol/#:~:text=If%20you%20do%20choose%20to

McAuliffe, L. (2022b, August 15). *Top 8 carnivore diet cheeses.* Doctor Kiltz. https://www.doctorkiltz.com/carnivore-diet-cheese/

Millard, E. (2022, July 27). *Will drinking salt water hydrate you more effectively than regular water?* Nike. https://www.nike.com/a/does-salt-water-aid-hydration

Munch-Andersen, T., Olsen, D. B., Søndergaard, H., Daugaard, Jens R., Bysted, A., Christensen, D. L., Saltin, B., & Helge, Jørn W. (2012). Metabolic profile in two physically active Inuit groups consuming either a western or a traditional Inuit diet.

International Journal of Circumpolar Health, *71*(1), 17342. https://doi.org/10.3402/ijch.v71i0.17342

Naqitarvik, R., Andersen, C. C., & Rayner-Canham, G. (2022). *Living on the edge: Some chemistry of the Inuit diet.* University of Waterloo. https://uwaterloo.ca/chem13-news-magazine/fall-2022-special-edition/feature/living-edge

Newman, T. (2022, October 31). *What's the deal with nitrites and nitrates?* Zoe. https://joinzoe.com/learn/cancer-risk-nitrites-nitrates

National Cancer Institute. (2022, April). Nitrate. U.S. Department of Health and Human Services, National Institutes of Health. https://progressreport.cancer.gov/prevention/

nitrate#:~:text=When%20taken
%20into%20the%20body

Pal, S., Woodford, K., Kukuljan, S., & Ho, S. (2015). Milk intolerance, beta-casein and lactose. *Nutrients*, *7*(9), 7285–7297. https://doi.org/10.3390/nu7095339

Parsons, J. (2019, March 22). *Cavemen's diet really did just consist of eating meat, researchers claim.* Metro. https://metro.co.uk/2019/03/22/cavemens-diet-really-just-consist-eating-meat-researchers-claim-8984543/

Pray, L. (2008). Discovery of DNA structure and function: Watson and Crick. *Nature Education*, *1*(1). https://www.nature.com/scitable/topicpage/discovery-of-dna-structure-and-function-watson-397/

Rabinowitch, I. M., Smith, F. C., Bazin, E. V., & Mountford, M. (1936). Metabolic Studies of Eskimos in the Canadian Eastern Arctic. *The Journal of Nutrition, 12*(4), 337–356. https://doi.org/10.1093/jn/12.4.337

Rehm, J. (2011). The risks associated with alcohol use and alcoholism. *Alcohol Research & Health: The Journal of the National Institute on Alcohol Abuse and Alcoholism, 34*(2), 135–143. https://www.ncbi.nlm.nih.gov/pmc/articles/PMC3307043/

Rinninella, E., Raoul, P., Cintoni, M., Franceschi, F., Miggiano, G. A. D., Gasbarrini, A., & Mele, M. C. (2019). What is the healthy gut microbiota composition? A changing ecosystem across age, environment, diet, and diseases. *Microorganisms, 7*(1), 14. https://doi.org/10.3390/microorganisms7010014

Roxby, P. (2010, September 17). *Recreating the caveman diet.* BBC News. https://www.bbc.com/news/health-11075437

Sakamoto, K., Nishizawa, H., & Manabe, N. (2012). [Behavior of pesticides in coffee beans during the roasting process]. *Journal of the Food Hygienic Society of Japan, 53*(5), 233–236. https://doi.org/10.3358/shokueishi.53.233

Saladino, P. (2021, January 11). *What to eat on a carnivore diet. Your carnivore diet meal plan!* Heart & Soil. https://heartandsoil.co/what-to-eat-on-a-carnivore-diet/

Saladino, P. (2022, September 8). *The carnivore diet: Start here.* Heart & Soil. https://heartandsoil.co/the-carnivore-diet-start-here/

Sanchez, K. (2020, November 7). *Carnivore diet: A beginner's guide to an all-meat diet.*

Chomps. https://chomps.com/
blogs/nutrition-sustainability-
news/carnivore-diet

Slattery, E. (n.d.). *Foods for
constipation.* Johns Hopkins
Medicine. https://
www.hopkinsmedicine.org/
health/wellness-and-prevention/
foods-for-constipation

Streit, L. (2019, May 16). *What is sole
water, and does it have benefits?*
Healthline. https://
www.healthline.com/nutrition/
sole-water

Teague, R., & McRae, R. (n.d.). *Ancient
DNA and Neanderthals.*
Smithsonian National Museum of
Natural History. https://
humanorigins.si.edu/evidence/
genetics/ancient-dna-and-
neanderthals

UC Davis. (2022, July 21). *Why it's
important for you to drink water
and stay hydrated.* https://

health.ucdavis.edu/blog/good-food/why-its-important-for-you-to-drink-water-and-stay-hydrated/2022/07

WebMD Editorial Contributors. (n.d.). Health benefits of sole water. WebMD. https://www.webmd.com/diet/health-benefits-sole-water

Wilde, O. (n.d.). *Everything in moderation, including moderation* [Quote]. Goodreads. https://www.goodreads.com/quotes/22688-everything-in-moderation-including-moderation

Woods, T. (2022, November 22. *What's the carnivore diet?—A beginner's guide (2023)* Carnivore Style. https://carnivorestyle.com/carnivore-diet/

Yamagata, K. (2018). Do coffee polyphenols have a preventive action on metabolic syndrome associated endothelial dysfunctions? An assessment of the current evidence. *Antioxidants*, *7*(2), 26. https://doi.org/10.3390/antiox7020026

Printed in Great Britain
by Amazon